Transfer Factors

Nature's State-of-the-Art Immune Fortifiers

RITA ELKINS, M.H.

WOODLAND PUBLISHING
Pleasant Grove, Utah

Woodland Publishing
P.O. Box 160
Pleasant Grove, Utah
84062
Visit us at our web site: www.woodlandbooks.com
or call us toll-free: (800) 777-2665

The information in this book is for educational purposes only and is not recommended as a means of diagnosing or treating an illness. All matters concerning physical and mental health should be supervised by a health practitioner knowledgeable in treating that particular condition. Neither the publisher nor the author directly or indirectly dispenses medical advice, nor do they prescribe any remedies or assume any responsibility for those who choose to treat themselves.

ISBN 1-58054-096-1
Printed in the United States of America

Contents

Acknowledgment

I would like to thank Dr. William Hennen, Ph.D., for his exhaustive research on transfer factors and for his expertise on pharmacological compounds and immune function. His thorough investigation and writings on the subject have brought transfer factors to the forefront of both conventional and complementary medicine.

TRANSFER FACTORS

Nature's State-of-the-Art Immune Fortifiers

"Transfer factors are small proteins that 'transfer' the ability to express cell-mediated immunity from immune donors to non-immune recipients."

Molecular Medicine, April 6, 2000

We Need Superb Immune Support

For over ten years, I have had the opportunity to investigate hundreds of natural compounds. I can honestly report that the compound I discuss in this booklet ranks as the most fascinating and promising among the natural "heavyweights." After 3,000 peer-reviewed studies and fifty years of research, transfer factor isolate supplements are finally available to the general public. The review of transfer factors contained in this booklet may be the most important health news you will ever see.

Transfer factor is a term you will undoubtedly be hearing about in your neighborhoods and communities. These factors are creating unprecedented interest in the world of both alternative and conventional therapies.

Transfer factors are not vitamins, minerals, herbs, hormones or drugs. Transfer factors contain nothing foreign, nothing toxic, or nothing counterproductive.

Their health potential is considered by many health experts to be the most exciting discovery in immunology and disease prevention to date. In assessing the enormous value of a transfer factor supplement for you or your family, consider the following questions:

- Do you get recurring colds and sore throats easily?
- Do you or other members of your family fight chronic infections?
- Does cancer run in your family?

- Would you like to make your family more disease resistant with advanced immune support for life?
- Would you like to shorten the duration of infections without becoming dependent on antibiotics?
- Would you like to investigate the possibilities of a supplement so advanced in the way it fights disease, it cannot be classified as a vitamin, herb, mineral or any other compound?

Transfer factors are turning the heads of health professionals everywhere. Why?

The key to future health is to strengthen our immune defenses. Before we do anything else, we need to target immunity. So, before you take a whole host of supplements to enhance your health, begin with immune support.

Dr. Richard Bennet, Ph.D., an immunologist and expert in infectious disease, has said, "It's in our ability to create a really healthy immune system, which I think represents the greatest potential in gains in human health in the world. If we can do something to make us all just a little bit more healthy, there's going to be less disease and less suffering."

One thing I have learned over the course of my own investigative research is that when it comes to health, we often put the cart before the horse. Clearly, we diminish the value of using alternative treatments to fight off infections after we get sick if we neglect to keep our immune machine in tip top shape when we're in between illnesses. Whether we will live a healthy or a debilitated life depends solely on the health of our immune system.

Out of all the natural immune builders available, transfer factor holds the most promise. Relatively new to the market, every consumer who wants that extra edge in wellness needs to become familiar with the remarkable properties of transfer factor. It has already exceeded expectations and is clearly ahead of its time.

Transfer Factor Isolate: Immune Booster Extraordinaire

Imagine an immune system alert enough to rapidly detect the presence of threatening infection and eradicate it before it has a chance to do real harm. Transfer factor can make this scenario possible through its superb ability to help develop a strong immune response.

> "Recurrent or chronic infections, even very mild colds, are signs that the immune system is weakened. Support of the immune system is perhaps the most important step in achieving resistance to disease and reducing susceptibility to colds, flus, and cancer."
>
> *Michael Murray, N.D., and Joseph Pizzorno, N.D.*
> (ENCYCLOPEDIA OF NATURAL MEDICINE)

Obtaining a pure transfer factor isolate is now possible through the perfection of a patented extraction process that has been in the works for years. Unlike herbs like echinacea or vitamins and minerals, these factors belong to a completely different category of dietary supplementation—an innovative and novel category.

Researchers at the Conrad D. Stephenson Laboratory for Research in Immunology in Denver, Colorado, who worked with people with immune weaknesses, have stated, "Transfer factors appear to offer a novel means of molecular immunotherapy for certain patients with defective cell-mediated immunity."

The Immune Wars

It is up to each of us individually to take the necessary steps to reinforce our immune system. Immune impairment has become a major concern. The use of compounds like transfer factor can significantly contribute to immune strength, which in turn determines the quality of our health and, ultimately, of our lives.

> ***Transfer factors can aid in the fight against the following conditions:***
>
> - viral infections
> - parasitic diseases
> - malignant diseases
> - mycobacterial diseases
> - fungal infections
> - autoimmune diseases
> - bacterial diseases
> - neurological diseases

Immune Imbalance: The Health Threat of the 21st Century

Every day, new studies are published that point to a malfunctioning immune system as the real culprit in conditions like heart disease, obesity, and multiple sclerosis. Our immune systems are letting us down. The more we learn, the more we realize that tuning up our immune systems is the best investment we can make for extended good health and longevity.

> ***Immune dysfunction may be the real cause of a variety of disorders usually linked to other factors.***

Scientists are discovering that diseases once thought to be unrelated to infectious invaders are really caused by microorganisms that either fail to trigger the proper immune response or overstimulate that response. One of these is a debilitating disease called multiple sclerosis.

A Common Bacteria Linked to MS

A startling report found in the July 1999 issue of *Annals of Neurology* reported that a common bacterium called *Chlamydia pneumoniae* was present in all the patients tested in the study with multiple sclerosis (MS). This bacteria is the same one that causes walking pneumonia. While MS has been classified as an autoimmune disorder in which the immune system's defense mechanisms mistakenly destroy the nerve coverings, new studies tell us that a bacteria may really be to blame.

Note: A viral link has also been discovered to MS. Recent data out of the National Institute of Neurological Disorders and Stroke suggests that a herpes virus found in 30 percent of people tested with MS may be linked to the disease.

In both of these scenarios, it is thought that the infectious agent remains dormant in nerve tissue until a flare up.

Weight and the Hidden Virus

Even gaining weight may be related to an immune system that's out of balance. Researchers at the Department of Nutrition and Food Science at Wayne State University in Detroit reported in

August of this year that increased fat stores have been linked to the presence of a virus. If a viral infection contributes to obesity, the

> *Transfer factor supplementation has had some dramatic success against nerve diseases that have a viral cause.*

first line of attack in any weight loss program should be to bring the immune system up to optimal levels of operation. All the diets and exercise in the world will ultimately fail if your weight gain is linked to the presence of viruses that promote the storage of fat, regardless of what you eat or how much you move.

Viruses and Bacteria Masquerade as Heart and Kidney Disease

In the August 2000 issue of the *American Journal of Medicine*, scientists reported that the hepatitis C virus can show up as a kidney infection or as heart disease. This year, Italian researchers at the Hospital of San Camillo in Rome reported that there is growing evidence that the immune system is involved in atherosclerosis. The same bacterium linked to MS (*Chlamydia pneumoniae*) may also be a culprit in heart disease as well. The health implications of these studies is staggering. Once again, if persistent infection is really causing heart disease, we've been on the wrong treatment track for decades.

> ***Transfer factor supplementation can "prime" the immune system, which may protect organs like the heart from infectious agents.***

Arthritis May Be the Result of a Joint Infection

It may come as a surprise to many, but some forms of arthritis occur after bouts with intestinal infections. In addition, Dutch scientists recently reported that chronic arthritis may have a bacteri-

> *"The daily stresses in our lives and simply living on this planet jeopardize and compromise optimal immune system function. Transfer factor will enhance your ability to respond to those challenges. Transfer factor is about staying healthy."*
>
> ***June Ferrari, N.D., Certified Nutrition Counselor***

al connection. In fact, if you suffer from rheumatoid arthritis, an autoimmune disease, your disease may have been triggered by a prior infection that may have overstimulated immune responses, which in this scenario, need suppressing.

Epilepsy Linked to Abnormal Immune System Cells

In 1997, a group of scientists looked at a total of 135 people with epilepsy. More than 80 percent of these people had one or more abnormalities in their cellular immune defenses. Some types of epilepsy may be caused by impaired immunity.

Transfer factor supplementation strengthens the cellular immune system and may be a valuable supplemental treatment to control epileptic seizures.

Alzheimer's Disease Linked to the Immune System

An article in a 1994 issue of *Progress in Drug Research* reported that Alzheimer's disease may be linked to an abnormal antibody response to a portion of nerve cells in the brain. This immune malfunction may destroy brain tissue associated with memory.

The Terrible Trio That Assaults the Immune System

1. Poor Nutrition

FACT: All forms of sugar (including honey) interfere with the ability of white blood cells to destroy bacteria. A report published in the *American Journal of Clinical Nutrition* stated that within thirty minutes of consuming four ounces of glucose, fructose, sucrose, honey or fruit juice, a 50 percent reduction in the ability of white blood cells to destroy foreign invaders occurs and can last for over five hours.

Trying to improve your health before targeting immune fitness is like putting the cart before the horse.

The average American ingests 150 grams of white sugar daily.

FACT: Suppressed immunity can come from even a minor deficiency of iron and selenium, two minerals that significant numbers of Americans are lacking. In addition, vitamin A deficiencies are common in children and can cripple immune functions.

FACT: Excessive fat intake impairs immunity. Elevated cholesterol levels can inhibit a number of immune functions including the ability of white blood cells to attack infectious organisms.

FACT: Obesity has been linked to weakened immune function. Overweight people have debilitated white blood cells.

2. Pollution

FACT: Hundreds of studies using accepted scientific methods have shown that many pesticides alter the immune system in experimental animals and make them more susceptible to disease.

The constant assault of stresses, such as the following, weaken our natural immune defenses.

- free radicals
- tobacco
- poor digestion
- bad fats
- international travel
- drug side effects
- day care
- alcohol
- aging
- sleep disorders
- weight-loss diets
- eating disorders
- antibiotic abuse
- additives

FACT: Pesticides reduce the numbers of white blood cells and disease-fighting lymphocytes, and impair lymphocytes' ability to respond to and kill bacteria and viruses.

FACT: A recent report published in *Environmental Pollution and Neuroimmunology* states that the combined influence of various factors such as chemical agents, radiation, and stress on the immune system may lead to immunodeficiency in the form of respiratory and inflammatory diseases.

3. Stress

FACT: Stress releases biochemicals that suppress immune function, putting us at higher risk for all types of infections.

FACT: How and what we think impacts immunity. New data reports that brain cells make immune chemicals.

FACT: Post-traumatic stress suffered after Hurricane Andrew lowered immune-killer cell counts in test subjects. Any life-changing event brings with it a form of post-traumatic stress, which can make us more susceptible to disease.

Antibiotic Resistance and the "Super Bugs"

"Bacterial resistance to antibiotics is a growing public health threat to the United States," says Richard Besser, M.D., of the CDC's respiratory disease branch.

Substances once thought to be miracle drugs are currently posing one of the most serious health threats we have faced in decades.

Current microorganisms that are becoming more resistant to antibiotics

- *Streptococcus pneumoniae*
- *Staphylococci*
- meningococcal infections
- mutant *E. coli*
- group A *Streptococci*
- *Pneumococcus*
- *Candida albicans*

Bacteria are now outwitting even our most potent antibiotics, creating a global threat of enormous proportions.

We all shudder at the thought of flesh-eating bacteria or penicillin-resistant strep bacteria, but even new drug formulas can hardly keep up. Some experts believe we are only one antibiotic away from a major epidemic of antibiotic-resistant bacteria.

If these antibiotic-resistant bacteria continue to evolve at the present rate, having a strong and fortified immune system may be your family's only defense against a whole host of life-threatening diseases.

March 11, 1998 issue of USA TODAY reported: "At least 70 percent of the bacteria that cause hospital-acquired infections are resistant to at least one antibiotic."

The Centers for Disease Control and Prevention (CDC) estimates that 100 million courses of antibiotics are provided by office-based doctors each year. In 1954, two million pounds of antibiotics were produced in the United States. Today, that figure exceeds fifty million pounds.

Some experts believe 20 to 50 percent of antibiotic prescriptions are unnecessary. Remember that antibiotics are only effective against bacteria. They are completely useless against the viruses that cause colds, flus and some sore throats.

Because of the misuse of antibiotics to treat common conditions like sinusitis, resistance to many antibiotics, even in the most common bacterial causes of upper respiratory infections, has risen to 40 to 50 percent in the last two decades.

Overusing these drugs can also cause yeast and fungal infections. Frequent use can compromise your immune system, stimulate allergies, damage organs, and even cause depression.

If Antibiotics Fail Us, What Then?

The simple answer to this question is to fortify the body's own defense team. Transfer factor supplementation is an excellent form of immune support.

First-Rate, First-Line Immune Defense

When your throat gets scratchy, you feel feverish, or you see a red welt developing around that tiny splinter, you are seeing the

> **Common Immune Foibles**
>
> When the immune system overreacts to an antigen such as pollen, an allergic reaction can result.
>
> When immune sensors misread antigens found on our own cells and attack, autoimmune disorders like lupus erythematosus or rheumatoid arthritis can develop.
>
> When the immune system fails to react properly to an outside invader, infections take hold.
>
> When the immune system fails to recognize the body's own cells after they become malignant, cancer can occur.

effects of a highly sophisticated immune defense strategy. Symptoms of a sickness tell us that our immune defenses have mounted a counterattack against whatever infectious agent has entered our body. In order to work well, our immune system must operate like a well-oiled machine.

Much like the workings of a sensitive radar, the immune system must recognize germs as foreign intruders and separate them from the body's own cells and molecules. Because it works on a molecular level, immune cells work as part of a highly complex and reactive system. The immune system's ability to respond properly determines our very health and survival.

When bacteria, viruses, fungi, toxins or cancer cells invade, the immune system springs into action, seeking out and eradicating the infectious enemy. Immune system agents are activated to neutralize potentially dangerous microbes. In addition, other immune cells act as messengers, releasing molecules that work to fine tune the whole process.

Whenever our immune system successfully foils an infection, it emerges stronger and better equipped to fight future health threats.

The Antigen Factor

All cells, including infectious invaders, carry identifiable antigens on their surface. An antigen is any substance that causes the immune system to produce antibodies. Much like individual fingerprints, these specific molecular signatures tell the immune system whether the cell is friend or foe. This is why transplanted organs are often attacked by the recipient's immune system. Their foreign antigen codes are translated as intruder cells so the immune system mounts its attack. It is estimated that our bodies can react to over 100 million different antigens.

While our immune system routinely sifts and sorts through trillions of cells and their antigen codes, it may be lacking as many as 50,000 specific antigen responses. Without immune awareness of those missing cellular imprints, we become more vulnerable to those specific invaders. In addition, keep in mind that many infectious agents routinely mutate, fooling the immune systems. This is why we can catch multiple colds and flus over the course of time.

We already possess our own innate storehouse of immune molecules called transfer factors that occupy our T lymphocytes. These factors enable the T cells of our immune system to set off immediate alarms when certain antigens are identified as undesirable. So, you can see why adding to our already existing stockpile of transfer factors would be a good thing.

The Key: A Maximized Immune Messaging System

Transferring the right information from one group of immune cells to another helps to prevent each of the four threats mentioned previously.

The right molecular messengers can instruct, coordinate, activate and suppress immune cells *according to need.*

We usually operate with information collected from our own immune experience or exposure, but we can do much better than that. Our immune system needs maximum access to molecular information whether it comes from our own internal data banks or whether it is imported from other sources. The point is that whether generated from within or from without, immune messenger molecules in the form of transfer factors all speak the same language.

Transfer Factors: Immune Teachers of the Three R's

When a microbial invader attacks, a healthy immune system must be proficient in the three R's:

RECOGNIZE — REACT — REMEMBER

To fight off disease and function at optimal levels, the immune system must do the following:

- Recognize a disease-causing organism for what it is.
- Organize and mount an attack to eradicate that organism.
- Remember the antigen signature of that organism so the next time it invades, an immediate response occurs.

Transfer factors provide a highly concentrated, immune messaging system, designed by nature to transfer critical immune programming from one individual to another. Transfer factors imprint on the infant immune system the recognition codes it needs to identify pathogens as hostile invaders.

Simply stated, transfer factors are tiny immune messenger molecules made up of a sequence of amino acids that impart immune signals between immune cells. In other words, transfer factors educate naive cells about a present or a potential danger.

Through a special and patented process, concentrated transfer factors can now be "lifted" out of cow colostrum, collected and offered in a pure, powerful, concentrated extract.

Transfer Factors Speed the Critical Recognition Stage

Did you know the time it takes to identify an invader is the time when we come down with the symptoms of an infection? It only stands to reason the sooner an invader is recognized, the shorter the duration of the illness.

An immature immune response can take ten to fourteen days to fully develop. In the meantime, you will feel the effects of "fighting off" an infection. Transfer factors can "induce" or speed up that recognition phase. A 1996 issue of *Biotherapy* reported that transfer factors can stimulate a response in less than twenty-four hours.

Clearly, if we add more transfer factors to our immune arsenal, the transfer of information from cell to cell is enhanced. You see, transfer factors work to teach new immune cells about old threats. As a result, we develop a stronger, more efficient immune system capable of fighting off constant assaults.

Transfer factors boost your immune system's ability recognize and respond to specific antigens. They are considered all-natural and work by "tutoring" your own immune system to identify infectious agents that attack your body every day.

> "What we discovered is something that's been there since the beginning of time, that we've overlooked because of the scientific blinders we had on . . . there's something in cow's colostrum that can make us healthier."
>
> *Richard Bennett, Ph.D.*

Transfer Factors Shorten Immune Response Time

The unique action of transfer factors helps expedite the immune system's response to a threat. How do transfer factors do it? The following illustrate how transfer factor speeds the immune system response.

- Transfer factors download extra information into human immune memory banks.
- Transfer factors provide our T lymphocyte cells a blueprint to follow to build a swift attack, cutting down the time they take to fight infection.
- Transfer factors provide immune markers to more quickly guide T cell reactions to an invader.
- Transfer factors help the immune system widen its storehouse of antibodies, which helps to expand immune memory to better remember and deal with future infections.

Where Do Transfer Factors Come From?

In humans, transfer factors from a mother's more experienced immune system pass to her baby via colostrum (the first milk that the offspring receives immediately after birth). Colostrum is packed with an army of immune components that pass to the newborn. In so doing, the new baby's immune system has the advantage of a much older one against millions of potential invaders. In addition, the immune tutors that come from the mother's colostrum train the infant's immune cells, so they can mount future defenses of their own.

Through colostrum, mother nature has provided a marvelous way for a baby's immature immune system to benefit from an older one that has already fought off thousands of infections. As a

> **Did You Know?**
> Calves who do not nurse from their mothers soon after birth will die within a few days from overwhelming infections caused by the most common organisms.

result, the infant is afforded protection and fortification in fighting off infections.

Through colostrum, the infant inherits the mother's immune data. Transfer factors, tiny molecular structures, are arguably the most valuable part of the colostrum.

The past notion that colostrum was only rich in nutrients and could be artificially replaced in formula led to a rapid rise in childhood allergies and a decrease in overall childhood health. Colostrum is so much more than a nutritious liquid.

Colostrum is Packed with Immune Builders

While scientists knew that colostrum contained antibodies made by the mother against infectious organisms, they only recently recognized that transfer factors are also present in this nutritious fluid and are just as important.

Transfer Factors Are Not Species Specific

We know now that transfer factors produced by a cow can work just as effectively in humans as they do in animals—something you cannot say about the antibody content of cow colostrum. In other words, transfer factors extracted from cow colostrum can give us the same type of advantage a newborn gets from its mother's first milk.

The ability to receive immune data transferred from the cow to the human has the potential to revolutionize the way we look at disease prevention in medicine.

Keep in mind that all mammals, including humans and cattle, come into constant contact with the same micro-organisms. Animals and humans alike live in the same microbial world, and all mammals have immune systems that work alike.

When a cow comes in contact with a bacteria or virus or a parasite, its immune system responds the same way we do. It recognizes the invader, identifies it, responds, and then remembers. These immune memories are subsequently encoded on tiny memory molecules called transfer factors.

Is Transfer Factor Supplementation Better than Cow's Colostrum?

1. Unlike the immunoglobulins (antibodies) found in cow colostrum, transfer factors are non-allergenic, whereas cow colostrum contains antibodies that can cause allergic reactions in some individuals.

2. Transfer factor isolates have been estimated to contain more than 200 individual factors. They are much more "factor full" or concentrated than colostrum supplements, which only contain small amounts of random factors. In other words, they contain the most powerful part of cow colostrum.

3. Transfer factor isolates are not species-specific. The human body will not reject them as foreign. Cow colostrum contains elements that may not be readily accepted in a human system.

4. To see significant effectiveness, a person would have to take an enormous amount of colostrum to equal the transfer factor punch found in an extracted product.

Through these tiny factors, we can actually borrow immune memory from a compatible source, the cow, which has already experienced hundreds of infectious organisms, so when we encounter any of these organisms as we inevitably do every day, we have an incredible advantage. Our immune forces skip the identification and recognition stage, which is the time we normally become ill, and go directly to the attack mode, or secondary stage of defense.

Differences between Cow Colostrum and Transfer Factor Extract

Cow colostrum naturally contains some random transfer factors but the overall "punch" of these factors pales in comparison to concentrated isolates of transfer factor. In other words, the ability to separate out transfer factors from the rest of cow colostrum results in a superior product. In addition, taking whole cow colostrum may cause an allergic reaction in those sensitive to cow's milk.

> "Other products advertise the inclusion of transfer factors, but none of them have been produced with an exclusive patented extraction process, which makes this product more varied and concentrated."
>
> **Kenneth Singleton, M.D.**

Who Discovered Transfer Factor?

In 1949, Dr. H. Sherwood Lawrence made a very significant discovery. In the process of studying tuberculosis, which was a major health threat at the time, he discovered an immune response could be transferred from a donor to a recipient through an injection of an extract of leukocytes (white blood cells). Further investigation led him to conclude that this immune extract must contain "factors" that made it possible to transfer the donor's immunity to the recipient. He called these molecules "transfer factors."

In 1989, two researchers completed what was to become a patented process for actually extracting transfer factors from cow colostrum, resulting in a concentrated form. The patent reference is U.S. Patent 4,816,563.

In 1999, the effectiveness and safety of transfer factor supplementation was validated by scores of clinical studies worldwide. Scientists are just beginning to grasp the profound implications of transfer factor therapy in determining the health of not only present, but future generations.

Dr. Gary Wilson and Dr. Greg Paddock successfully completed a myriad of tests to win USDA approval for their transfer factor technology. It is this unique, patented technology that makes it possible to isolate or to separate transfer factors from cow colostrum. Through this extraction technique, pure transfer factors can be collected from the cow's first milk, dried and then encapsulated for human consumption.

Is Transfer Factor Backed by Scientific Data?

To date, over 3,000 clinical studies and papers have been published on transfer factors. Scores of international, well-respected scientists and physicians have established the effectiveness and safety of transfer factors. Over the last fifty years, an estimated

$40 million has been spent on research, and study data strongly suggests that transfer factors offer extraordinary immune benefits. Well documented and scientifically validated, transfer factors have emerged as profoundly important tools to health maintenance worldwide.

Recently, a symposium on transfer factors was held in Italy where transfer factor researcher Dr. D. Viza spoke about the potential of transfer factor in an era when "the toll of several diseases, such as cancer, continues to rise and the pathogenesis of AIDS remains elusive."

Anytime we can boost the action of natural killer (NK) cells (our immune cells that seek out and destroy foreign invaders), we greatly enhance our ability to fight disease.

In February of 1999, the *Journal of the American Nutraceutical Association* published a selection of 196 natural products or combinations, selected from over 400 products tested. Forty-four products were found to significantly enhance natural killer cell activity. The most powerful of these was able to increase natural killer cell action by 48.6 percent.

Transfer factor from colostrum was tested individually and raised natural killer cell activity by an extraordinary 103 percent above baseline values.

If that wasn't impressive enough, when transfer factor was combined with a variety of other natural compounds that also support immunity, it increased natural killer cell activity by 248 percent above baseline values!

What do these test studies suggest? Simply stated, these unprecedented numbers elevate transfer factor to the top of the nutraceutical list of immune boosters.

The Implications

Anyone who is prone to illness, i.e., colds, sore throats, ear infections, sinusitis, influenza, boils, chronic fatigue, parasites, fungal infections, tumors, compromised immunity, gum infections, etc., needs to take a serious look at the benefits of transfer factors. Transfer factors outperformed leading natural immune boosters with wide margins, suggesting that transfer factor isolates offer something more than other immune boosting compounds currently available.

OVERACTIVE IMMUNE DISORDERS		
• allergies	• asthma	• urticaria (hives)
• eczema	• rhinitis	• allergies
AUTOIMMUNE DISEASES		
• multiple sclerosis	• Type I diabetes	• psoriasis
• lupus	• scleroderma	• ITP
• rheumatoid arthritis		
INFLAMMATORY DISORDERS		
• fibromyalgia	• Crohn's disease	• celiac disease
• irritable bowel	• ulcerative colitis	
UNDERACTIVE IMMUNE DISORDERS		
• infection	• HIV	• hepatitis B/C
• cancer	• shingles	• sinusitis
• tuberculosis	• chronic fatigue	• cold and flu

Autoimmune Diseases and Transfer Factor

Transfer factors can also suppress an overactive immune system involved in autoimmune diseases. If your immune system is too weak, you become susceptible to bacterial, viral, fungal and parasitic infections. If your immune system is overactivated, you become susceptible to autoimmune diseases, where the immune system attacks human tissue it mistakenly identifies as foreign such as lupus, Type 1 diabetes, rheumatoid arthritis, psoriasis, etc.

Transfer Factors for Overactive Immune Functions

Transfer factor isolates contains immune modulators made up of both *activators* and *suppressors*, which not only serve as a wake-up call to immunity, but also help to normalize and balance an overly aggressive immune system as seen in cases of, chronic fatigue, rheumatoid arthritis, multiple sclerosis and lupus.

In 1976, transfer factor pioneer H. Sherwood Lawrence began investigating the potential of transfer factor for people with

Enhancement of NK Cell Activity By Natural Products

Compound Tested	% Rise over Baseline
Noni (*Morinda citrifolia*)	15%
Aloe Vera Concentrate	15%
Herbal Formula with Garlic	21%
Bovine Colostrum	23%
Cordyceps Formula	28%
Shiitake Mushroom	42%
Echinacea	43%
Polysaccharide Formula	48%
Transfer Factor	103%
Transfer Factor Combination	248%

Source: Life Extension Institute, 1999

autoimmune disorders. Today, transfer factor can be used to treat various autoimmune conditions because it serves to modulate and normalize immune response.

Dr. William Hennen, Ph.D., an expert in pharmacological compounds and author of *Transfer Factor* and *Enhanced Transfer Factor*, has done extensive research on the therapeutic benefits of these immune molecules. The following information on a few diseases and disorders that can be treated with transfer factors comes from his exhaustive investigations:

Juvenile rheumatoid arthritis. Japanese researchers found that transfer factor supplementation was used with good success in cases of juvenile rheumatoid arthritis that were unresponsive to even high doses of steroids and immunosuppressants.

Juvenile diabetes mellitus. In 1996, scientists reported that both the inducer and the suppressor actions of transfer factor

> Immune imbalance underlies many chronic illnesses. Because transfer factor can function as an immune modulator, it can help to restore immune system balance in many types of clinical situations.
>
> *Kenneth Bock, MD*

preparations may have contributed to its long-lasting, anti-diabetic effect in studies. This is good news for anyone with Type I diabetes.

Atopic dermatitis. Thirty test subjects with moderate to severe atopic dermatitis were treated with transfer factor supplementation and significant improvement was seen in the four major symptoms of this painful skin disorder.

Transfer Factor for Children

FACT: Children have immature immune systems and are prone to infections that easily spread in day-care and school settings.

FACT: Children often eat diets high in sugar and low in nutrients necessary to support immunity.

FACT: Children spread infections rapidly in schools and day-care centers.

FACT: Ear infections are increasing with heavy reliance on antibiotic drugs that are rapidly failing to control the recurring infections.

FACT: Antibiotic overuse in children causes compromised immunity and the development of antibiotic-resistant bacteria.

Transfer factors are benign, completely safe, tasteless and easy to take. Children seem to especially benefit from transfer factor supplementation. These factors are usually placed in a benign,

Why Children Need Transfer Factor

- Transfer factor saves thousands of dollars in medical costs.
- Transfer factor helps to halt the vicious cycle of sore throats, colds and ear infections.
- Transfer factor helps to stop the overuse of antibiotics and safely strengthens a child's immune system
- Transfer factor can be safely given to infants as young as three weeks old

> *"I have been running a clinical trial in my pediatric practice for twelve months. In an aged-matched review of transfer factor users, we have seen 74 percent less reported illness and 84 percent less use of antibiotics. I've been amazed, but not surprised, because I've seen the research on transfer factor."*
>
> **David Markowitz, M.D.**

completely safe and tasteless carrier substance that can easily be added to formula or food.

Dr. David Markowitz, a pediatrician who practices in Maine has just finished a review of his first twelve months' experience with transfer factor supplementation. The study found that eighty-eight children who used transfer factor isolates daily at the recommended doses for six or more months showed a 74 percent reduction in reported illness and an 84 percent reduction in antibiotic use. Using any measure, these are very significant results. Of equal importance is the fact that no side effects were reported. In addition, Dr Markowitz emphasized that initial results indicate that over $25,000 was saved by the group using transfer factor supplements in medical care, office visits, and drug costs.

Transfer Factor for Childhood Ailments

Autism

Autism may be caused by exposure to a virus, especially rubella, which causes a form of measles. Many researchers believe that the battle between a very young and immature immune system and the virus causes the development of autism. In addition, some studies suggest that true autism may be an abnormal reaction to a live virus vaccine in certain susceptible children that have immature immune systems. Researchers have found that autistic children often suffer from weak immune systems. Of twenty-two autistic children treated with transfer factor supplements, twenty-one responded favorably. Ten of the children improved both emotionally and mentally, enough that they were able to enter mainstream schools.

Kenny's Story

Kenny is a twenty-year-old young man who contracted HIV from contaminated transfusions as part of his hemophilia treatment. He had been on retroviral therapy, which did not seem to be effective and caused him to suffer significant side effects. Kenny started taking high doses of a transfer factor isolate daily as part of his treatment plan. He has remained infectious-disease free while on TF, and he has a **zero** viral count. Although Kenny is certainly not cured, he believes his dramatic improvement is due to transfer factor therapy, and he is spreading the word.

Cancer

Dr. Markowitz has also seen the value of transfer factor therapy for an eleven-year-old boy with lymphoblastic leukemia. After chemotherapy and a bone marrow transplant, he still experienced a relapse, and his leukemia actually became more severe. Enhanced transfer factor supplements were used in combination with chemotherapy treatments, and the results have been very encouraging. Supplementing chemotherapy with transfer factors appeared to support the boy's immune system and prevent the infections that usually take hold during treatment. His doctors believe that his supplementation with transfer factors most likely spared him the life-threatening complications of infectious disease and apparently improved his tolerance of a very toxic course of chemotherapy.

Transfer Factor: A Boon for the Elderly

When it comes to beefing up deteriorating immune systems, transfer factor can turn back the clock. Consider the fact that hundreds of studies tell us that immune vigor declines with age contributing to increased infection and even death. If transfer factor supplementation can help the immature immune systems of children fight disease, it can exert a similar beneficial action in the elderly.

Older individuals are susceptible to yeast infections, bladder infections, mental disorders and influenza, which accounts for thousands of deaths annually among older communities.

Supplementing a good diet fortified with additional vitamins and minerals for older individuals could help prevent devastating infections, which are costly both in terms of money and of misery.

The Viral Vice and Transfer Factors

It is also so vitally important to understand that medical science offers little in the way of viral treatment. Transfer factors can help to protect us against viral infections like various strains of herpes and influenza. Dr. William Hennen's research points to Chinese and European studies that have found a dramatic drop in the duration and recurrence of herpes infections. What this means is that transfer factor can not only treat existing herpes, but also prevent future breakouts as well. This same action may apply to other viral infections like chronic fatigue, influenza and bronchitis.

Epstein-Barr and Chronic Fatigue Syndrome

Dr. Hennen cites a study in which three out of six patients treated with transfer factor for Epstein-Barr virus (which causes chronic fatigue), showed significant improvement. Other viruses such as chicken pox, measles and even the common cold can be treated with transfer factor. Another study referenced by Dr. Hennen revealed that transfer factor supplementation in two patients with chronic fatigue resulted in total remission, and seven showed dramatic improvement.

Herpes

Herpes is a viral infection that is difficult to treat. Dr. Hennen refers to a clinical trial of thirty-seven patients with herpes in which 62 percent showed marked improvement in either a recurrence or in the duration of herpes, going from twelve herpes incidences per year to 3.5 with transfer factor supplementation. Another study published in a 1996 issue of *Biotherapy* concluded that transfer factor treatment selectively affects immune cell production against the herpes simplex virus.

Hepatitis

Dr. Hennen also states that the use of transfer factors has been

> ***"All our cancer patients are on transfer factor. It really buoys the immune system up. You're looking at a product that is truly revolutionary. I think we have a duty to get the word out, to make people healthier, and to enjoy life more. My patients are doing it; we need more people doing it."***
>
> *Dr. Duane Townsend, Gynecologist & Oncologist, Salt Lake City, Utah*

shown to be highly effective in treating hepatitis. He points out that it has been reported that six million Chinese currently take hepatitis-specific transfer factor to prevent outbreaks of this prevalent disease.

Fibromyalgia

Although the cause of fibromyalgia, (a chronic muscuoloskeletal disease) remains unknown, anecdotal evidence exists that transfer factor therapy combined with other natural agents such as magnesium and malic acid works to ease symptoms.

Cancer

FACT: One in every three Americans will develop cancer. 1.2 million cancer cases are diagnosed every year in this country, and that number is going up, not down. Of these, six of ten people will die within five years.

FACT: One in every four deaths (over 500,000 each year) is attributable to cancer, and the rate is rising. The good news is that the National Cancer Institute estimates that over 75 percent of all cancer cases are preventable.

FACT: According to some experts at the National Cancer Institute, we are losing our battle with cancer because we've been on the wrong track. Prevention rather than cure should become our new emphasis.

What is cancer? It is a disease characterized by the uncontrolled growth of abnormal cells permitted to reproduce due to extensive immune collapse. Cancer is allowed to grow because our immune surveillance system falls asleep.

Our immune watch guards single out, identify and destroy carcinogenic agents that enter the body daily. Immune cells such as B-lymphocytes produce antibodies designed to attack and eradicate malignant cells, and a variety of immune chemicals keep tumors in check.

Given the multifaceted defense strategy of our immune system, it is remarkable that in some people, cancer cells grow without any detection. Why? Because people with faulty immune responses are at a much higher risk of developing cancer.

Because many of us cannot avoid exposure to pollution, pesticides, additives, ultra-violet rays, etc., it is crucial that we boost our natural immune defenses to protect us against cancer.

Transfer Factor as a Support to Chemotherapy

Cancer patients who are undergoing chemotherapy or radiation, which greatly weaken the immune system, can greatly benefit from taking transfer factor supplementation. Transfer factor supplementation serves to protect the body from "opportunistic" infections, which often occur during these treatments.

Dr. Duane Townsend, former director of gynecologic oncology at LDS Hospital in Salt Lake City, puts all of his cancer patients on transfer factor treatments to boost their immune systems' abilities to respond to any health challenges.

Both Japanese and Chinese clinical studies found that the immunosuppression that results from chemotherapy can be prevented by using transfer factor isolates. Keep in mind that the elimination of dying or dead cancer cells is monitored by the immune system. Italian, Japanese and American studies tell us that the use of transfer factor isolates to boost immune function after surgery significantly improves the chances of a cancer-free future.

> "For cancer to start and then continue growing, it must outmaneuver the many long arms of your immune defenses. The immune system is both your first and last defense against cancer."
>
> *John Bailar, M.D., Ph.D., former editor-in-chief of the* Journal of the National Cancer Institute

Bacterial Infections and Transfer Factor

In his research, Dr. William Hennen refers us to studies that suggest transfer factor supplementation may slow the rate at which bacteria grows, which then permits the immune system added time in which to mount an attack. In other words, this window of time allows for the production of specific antibodies needed to win the bacterial war.

Bladder infections

Dr. William Hennen, a biochemist and expert in transfer factor therapy and author of *Transfer Factor,* has stated:

"A woman suffering from chronic bacterial cystitis (bladder infection) who took a transfer factor preparation designed to treat both candida and cytomegalovirus found that her recurrence rate was reduced to less than 15 percent of her previous suffering."

Salmonella

Salmonella is the organism that is responsible for a great many cases of food poisoning. Dr. Hennen, in his book *Transfer Factor,* tells us that scientists at the Department of Microbiology, Immunology and Animal Hygiene, at the University of Veterinary Medicine, in Kosice, Czechoslovakia studied the effect of transfer factor therapy in calves infected with salmonella. They found that the earlier these calves received the transfer factor, the better they dealt with the salmonella. He also points out that another study reported that using specific transfer factor preparations inhibited the ability of the salmonella organism to penetrate tissue.

Did You Know?

The findings on bacterial infections strongly support the notion of taking transfer factor supplements on a daily basis to "get a jump" on bacterial invasion.

Fungal Infections and Transfer Factor Therapy

Regarding fungal infections caused by *Candida albicans*, Dr. Hennen cites studies showing that the sooner transfer factor is given, the better the result. He reminds us that mycobacteria, which are fungus-like bacteria, have also been successfully treated with transfer factors. This class of bacteria include tuberculosis, which has reemerged in this country over the last few years.

Parasitic Infections and Transfer Factor

Dr. Hennen also stresses that transfer factor isolates have been successfully used to treat a number of parasitic diseases including cryptosporidiosis, which took the lives of forty people in Milwaukee when it contaminated drinking water supplies.

Transfer Factor for Better Overall Health

If you believe that waiting until you get sick and then taking action is the only way to confront illness, your health price tag may be exorbitant. Taking control of immune health before a crisis occurs is by far the better way to go. Most of us wait to "catch" something before we give our immune system extra help. All of us can get a jump on illness by dealing disease a knock-out punch before it strikes.

Remember that every human being houses a multitude of bacteria, viruses and even malignant cells that never pose a threat because a well-operating immune system is doing its job.

It is when we let our immune defenses break down that the risk of serious illness presents itself. There is no magic bullet in the treatment of disease, as we have seen in the case of antibiotic abuse. Therefore, fortifying our immune systems on a day to day basis is the best way to protect our families and us from the threat of pathogens, poor diet, pollution, and stress. We must build up our natural resistance to disease rather than rely on drugs after we get sick, drugs that not only come with a whole host of side effects, but may ultimately fail us as well.

Take Transfer Factor Every Day

Research confirms that transfer factor supplementation helps to

> "Dietary supplementation may help us to attain an immunological advantage over invading microbes and invasive cancers."
>
> *William J. Hennen, Ph.D.*

protect the immune system, so it can protect us from disease threats linked to the following:

- international travel
- nursing homes
- pollution
- stress
- camping
- hospitals
- additives
- new bacteria
- daycare
- workplaces
- carcinogens
- potent viruses

Studies strongly suggest that taking transfer factor supplements before an infection has a chance to take hold gives the recipient the best chance to overcome that infection more rapidly.

In addition, at the first sign of sickness, stepping up the dose of a transfer factor supplement or using it in combination with other immune-boosting compounds provides an optimal therapeutic effect.

Safety of Transfer Factor in Supplement Form

Transfer factor supplementation has an excellent safety record. No adverse side effects associated with transfer factor supplements have been reported, even when given in high doses both orally and intravenously over long periods of time. Transfer factor supplements are safe for everyone from infants to the elderly. Placed in carrier agents, oral supplements are easy to take, tasteless and well accepted by anyone regardless of age. Keep in mind that since 1949, transfer factors have been studied extensively. The overwhelming consensus is that transfer factors taken in supplement form, can relieve suffering and do so in a perfectly safe way.

Who Can Take Transfer Factor?

Transfer factor is safe and effective for men, women and children of all ages.

Even Pets Can Benefit From Transfer Factor

Pets are just as susceptible to infection as we are. Using transfer factor therapy for pets is an excellent way to fortify animal immunity and health. As mentioned, the transfer factors extracted from cow colostrum are not species specific. Dogs, cats, horses, etc., can benefit from their immune codes as well as humans can. Because transfer factors are so safe, they offer a convenient way to protect your pet against harmful microbial threats. Transfer factor supplements are especially beneficial for animals who have been injured, are old, or seem prone to certain types of infectious diseases. They have been used in dogs, cats, horses and other mammals.

Is Transfer Factor Allergenic?

Remember that transfer factor concentrates do not contain the large proteins that are responsible for milk allergies. Look for transfer factor products that are obtained from high quality milk-producing herds in the United States that are strictly controlled to ensure excellent quality and safety. The patented process on record in which lactose and large milk proteins (proteins that cause milk allergies) are removed has been proven effective in producing a high-quality transfer factor isolate.

Enhancing Transfer Factor through Diet

Although transfer factor isolate alone has extraordinary properties, adding certain immune-booting phytochemicals, vitamins and minerals can make a good thing even better. Clearly, a pure transfer factor extract should be the basic building block for superior immune function, but adding complimentary compounds makes for a multifaceted immune supplement. In other words, this broadens the immune shield of transfer factors through the mutual action of selected immune-friendly substances. Listed below are several natural compounds that strengthen the immune.

Cordyceps Sinensis

Highly prized by the Chinese as an impressive herbal immune tonic, this fungus has been tested in over 2,000 subjects.

Considered extremely safe, this herbal compound increases a variety of immune actions by boosting immune chemicals such as interleukin-1 and 2 and boosting the count of helper-T and natural killer cells to fortify and expand the immune system's ability to respond to invaders (infectious, carcinogenic etc). Of equal importance in that *Cordyceps sinensis* also suppresses inappropriate immune reactions as seen in autoimmune diseases and has anti-tumor properties as well.

Beta-Glucans

Complex polysaccharides present in astragalus, maitake and coriolus mushrooms have the unique ability to act as "immunomodulators" and are being researched for their potential role in AIDS and cancer. Current studies indicate that at the very least these compounds can prevent white blood cell numbers from falling in persons given chemotherapy and radiotherapy, and work to elevate antibody levels in healthy persons. Beta-glucans are considered the workhorse of the immune activating polysaccharides and are well absorbed when taken orally. They are currently under investigation as a supportive tool for HIV infection.

Echinacea

Echinacea stimulates the production of immune natural killer cells and destroys a broad range of disease-causing bacteria. Echinacea can be a boon to elderly individuals who are particularly susceptible to bacterial infections. A new study conducted by scientists at McGill University in Montreal, Canada showed that two weeks of supplementation with echinacea rejuvenated the production and action of immune killer cells even in animals of advanced age. In addition, several other studies have concluded that echinacea taken orally stimulates the function of a variety of immune cells, particularly natural killer cells.

Berberine-containing Herbs

Herbs like goldenseal and goldenthread contain a powerful alkaloid called berberine, which also has natural antibiotic action. This year, scientists from the Biotechnology Center at Tufts

University in Medford, Massachusetts reported that berberine inhibited the growth of a very resistant strain of staphylococcus. Staph infections are difficult to treat by any standards. In addition, an article in the April, 2000 issue of *Alternative Medicine Review* stated that berberine extracts have significant antimicrobial activity against a variety of organisms, including bacteria, viruses, and fungi. Berberine-containing herbs top the list for bacterial diarrhea, intestinal parasites, and for bladder and eye infections.

Mannans

Mannans (specifically acemannan) are a carbohydrate extracted from the gel of the aloe vera leaf. This compound is thought to make aloe gel so healing for burns and other skin disorders. Studies show that acemannan increases the number and killing capacity of T lymphocytes by almost 50 percent. It also has significant anti-tumor activity and can help prevent the replication of viruses in the body. Acemannan is one of a few plant extracts used in people with AIDS. Studies confirm that it has significant value for bacterial, viral, and fungal infections.

DID YOU KNOW?

Transfer factor in isolate form alone and transfer factors in combination with other compounds increased immune potency by stimulating natural killer cell activity more than any other natural supplement on the market.

IP6

Also known as inositol hexaphosphate or phytic acid (IP6), this compound is found in legumes and the bran portion of several grains. The reason that high-fiber diets are considered anti-cancerous may be due to this very phytochemical. Several laboratory tests have confirmed that IP6 has impressive anti-cancer actions and in 1992, a patent was obtained to mix IP6 with inositol. IP6 is rapidly absorbed and is one of the most impressive anti-cancer compounds found in nature.

Zinc

Zinc supplements have been reported to considerably increase immune function. This effect may be especially important in the elderly.

Vitamin A and Beta Carotene

Vitamin A plays an important role in immune system function and helps mucous membranes, including those in the lungs, resist invasion by microorganisms. Beta-carotene and other carotenoids boost immune cell numbers and activity in both animal and human research. Placebo-controlled research has confirmed the positive benefits of beta-carotene supplements in increasing numbers of some white blood cells and enhancing cancer-fighting immune functions.

Vitamin C

Vitamin C stimulates the immune system by enhancing interferon levels and boosting the activity of certain immune cells. In controlled reports studying people doing heavy exercise, cold frequency was reduced an average of 50 percent with vitamin C supplements ranging from 600 to 1,000 mg per day.

Vitamin E

Vitamin E enhances some aspects of immune cell activity especially in the elderly. A combination of antioxidant vitamins A, C, and E significantly improved immune cell number and activity compared to placebo in a group of hospitalized elderly.

Thymic Factors

The thymus gland produces a complex array of factors that

work together to transform immature lymphocytes (white blood cells) into T cells. Two decades ago, a key thymic protein was discovered and isolated. This protein actually programs T4 helper cells in the immune system to seek out an invading pathogen and gives the go-ahead to T8 killer cells to search and destroy disease organisms. A patented process has been developed to grow this specific protein for commercial use in supplement form.

Glutamine

This amino acid is important for healthy immune system function. Liquid diets high in glutamine have been reported to help critically ill people recover more rapidly. One double blind study giving athletes who were prone to respiratory infections glutamine reported 81 percent without subsequent infection compared to 49 percent in the placebo group.

Lactobacillus acidophilus

This supplement helps replace friendly bacteria in the gastrointestinal tract that may help protect the body from potentially harmful organisms that reside in the intestine and can cause infection. Infectious diarrhea in children has been successfully reduced with acidophilus supplementation.

Conclusion

Transfer factors could be the most exciting discovery in immunology to date. As the 21st century unfolds, these tiny molecules will hold the key to health and well being. If you are interested in keeping up with the latest technology in health maintenance, transfer factors should top your list of natural supplements for the 21st century.

Glossary

Antibodies: Large protein molecules that bind to an antigen initiating a cascade of events that will eventually destroy the antigen organism or substance.

Antigen: Any substance that enters the body and causes the production of specific antibodies to fight against it.

Autoimmune disorder: Abnormal activity of the immune system in which antibodies are produced against the body's own tissue rather than a foreign invader.

B Cells: Immune cells that produce antibodies.

Cell-mediated Immunity: Immune actions not influenced by antibodies that build up resistance to disease-causing organisms.

Colostrum: The first milk of mammals that is initially consumed by the suckling offspring and contains nutrients, antibodies and transfer factor molecules.

Eosinophils (and Basophils): White blood cells that secrete histamine and other compounds in allergic reactions and also work to break down antigen-antibody substances.

Immunoglobulins: Another term for antibodies.

Interferon: A powerful immune-boosting compound that is made in cells to fight off viruses and malignant cells.

Lymph Nodes and Vessels: Components of the immune system that collect and disperse fluid called lymph, which is filtered and returned to the blood.

Lymphocyte: A white blood cell that is found in the lymph nodes.

Macrophages: Monocytes that live in lymph, spleen and liver tissues and consume foreign matter and infectious invaders.

Monocytes: White blood cells that collect debris after infections.

Neutrophils: White blood cells that surround and consume disease organisms and dead tissue.

T Cells: A type of lymphocyte that is controlled by the thymus gland. Controls many immune functions. Helper T cells boost white blood cell activity, suppressor T cells inhibit their mechanisms and killer T cells attack and destroy foreign invaders.

Thymus Gland: The primary immune system organ that produces T cells and cell-mediated immunity.

White Bloods Cells: A group of several types of blood cells that include eosinophils, basophils, monocytes and lymphocytes.

References

Alvarez-Thull L and Kirkpatrick CH "Profiles of cytokine production in recipients of transfer factors" Biotherapy (1996) 9(1-3):55-9.

Anderson R "The immunostimulatory, anti-inflammatory an anti-allergic properties of ascorbate" Advanced Nutrition Research (1984)6:19–45.

Anderson R et al "Vitamin C and cellular immune functions. Protection against hypochlorous acid-mediated inactivation of glyceraldehyde-3-phosphate dehydrogenase and ATP generation in human leukocytes as a possible mechanism of ascorbate-mediated immunostimulation" Annals of the New York Academy of Science (1990)587:34-48.

Bengmark S. "Immunonutrition: role of biosurfactants, fiber, and probiotic bacteria" Nutrition (1998)14:585–94.

Borysov VA et al "The adjuvant and specific activity of transfer factors to Candida albicans" Fiziol Zh (1998) 44(4):3-9.

Boucheix Cl et al "Activity of animal transfer factor in man" Lancet, (1977) 198-199.

Chandra RK "Nutrition and the immune system: an introduction" American Journal of Clincal Nutrition (1997) 66:460–63S.

Chew BP "Role of carotenoids in the immune response" Journal of Dairy Science (1993) 76:2804–11.

De la Fuente et al "Immune function in aged women is improved by ingestion of vitamins C and E" Canadian Journal of Physiological Pharmacology (1998)76:373–80.

Dhurandhar NV "Increased adiposity in animals due to a human virus" International Journal of Obesity and Related Metabolic Disorders (2000 Aug)24(8):989-96.

Duchateau J et al "Influence of oral zinc supplementation on the lymphocyte response to mitogens of normal subjects" American Journal of Clinical Nutrition (1981)34:88–93.

Dumonde DC et al "Eleventh International Congress on Transfer Factors" March 1-4, 1999, Monterrey, Nuevo Leon, Mexico Journal of Interferon Cytokine Research (2000 April) 20(4):439-41.

Famularo G "Infections, atherosclerosis, and coronary heart disease Annals of the Italian Medical Institute (2000 Apr-Jun) 15(2):144-55.

Fernandes CF et al "Therapeutic role of dietary lactobacilli and lactobacillic fermented dairy products" (FEMS Micro Rev) (1987):46:343–56.

Fortes C et al "The effect of zinc and vitamin A supplementation on the immune response in an older population" Journal of the American Geriatric Society (1998)46:19–26.

Fraker PJ et al "The dynamic link between the integrity of the immune system and zinc status" Journal of Nutrition (2000 May)130(5S Suppl):1399S-406S.

Fujisawa T et al "Randomized controlled trial of transfer factor immunochemotherapy as an adjunct to surgical treatment for primary adenocarcinoma of the lung" Japanese Journal of Surgery (1984) 14(6): 452-8.

Griffiths RD "Outcome of critically ill patients after supplementation with glutamine. Nutrition" (1997)13:752–54.

Han SN et al Immunology (2000 Aug)100(4):487-93.

Hennen, William J. Transfer Factor (Woodland, Pleasant Grove Utah: 1998).

Hennen, William J. Enhanced Transfer Factor (Woodland, Pleasant Grove, Utah: 2000) .

Herbert TB and Cohen S "Stress and immunity in humans: a meta-analytic review" Psychosomatic Medicine (1993 Jul-Aug)55(4):364-79.

"The influence of industrial environmental pollution on the immune system. New ideas of immunorehabilitation " in th. International. Conference on Environmental Pollution & Neuroimmunology 1995 - p.9.

Ironson G et al "Posttraumatic stress symptoms, intrusive thoughts, loss, and immune function after Hurricane Andrew" Psychosomatic Medicine (1997Mar-Apr) 59(2):128-41.

Jones C et al "Randomized clinical outcome study of critically ill patients given glutamine-supplemented enteral nutrition" Nutrition (1999)15:108–15.

Kazi N et al "Immunomodulatory effect of beta-carotene on T lymphocyte subsets in patients with resected colonic polyps and cancer" Nutrition and Cancer (1997)28:140–45.

Kelley DS and Daudu PA "Fat intake and immune response" Prog Food Nutr Sci (1993)17:41–63.

Kemeny ME and Gruenewald TL "Affect, cognition, the immune system and health" Progressive Brain Research (2000)122:291-308.

Kemeny ME and Gruenewald TL. "Psychoneuroimmunology update" Seminar on Gastrointestinal Disease (1999)10:20–29.

Keplinger H. "Oxindole alkaloids having properties stimulating the immunologic system and preparation containing same" US Patent no. 5,302,611, April 12, 1994.

Kirkpatrick CH "Activities and characteristics of transfer factors"

Biotherapy (1996)1-3:13-6.
Kirkpatrick CH "Biological response modifiers. Interferons, interleukins, and transfer factor" Annals of Allergy (1989) 62(3): 170-6.
Kirkpatrick CH Structural nature and functions of transfer factors. Ann N Y Acad Sci (1993 Jun 23) 685:362-8.
Kirkpatrick CH "Therapeutic potential of transfer factor" [editorial] New. England Journal of Medicine (1980)14; 303(7): 390-1.
Kirkpatrick CH "Transfer factors: identification of conserved sequences in transfer factor molecules" Molecular Medicine (2000 April) 6(4):332-41.
McMeeking A et al" A controlled trial of bovine dialyzable leukocyte extract for cryptosporidiosis in patients with AIDS" Journal of Infectious Diseases (1990) 161: 108-12.
Melchart D et al "Immunomodulation with echinacea—a systematic review of controlled clinical trials" Phytomedicine (1994)1:245–54.
Melchart D et al "Results of five randomized studies on the immunomodulatory activity of preparations of echinacea" Journal of Alternative and Complementary Medicine (1995)1:145–60.
Meydani SN et al "Vitamin E supplementation enhances cell-mediated immunity in healthy elderly subjects" American Journal of Clinical Nutrition (1990)52:557–63.
Meydani SN et al "Vitamin E supplementation and in vivo immune response in healthy elderly subjects: a randomized controlled trial" Journal of the American Medical Association (1997)277:1380–86.
Mikula I et al "Dialyzable leukocyte extract used in the prevention of Salmonella infection in calves" Veterinary Immunology Immunopathology (1992 Apr) 32(1-2):113-24.
Nanba H "Antitumor activity of orally administered 'D-fraction' from maitake mushroom (Grifola frondosa)" Journal of Naturopathic Medicine (1993) 4:10–15.
Neequaye J et al "Specific transfer factor with activity against Epstein-Barr virus reduces late relapse in endemic Burkitt's lymphoma" Anticancer Research (1990) 10(5A): 1183-7.
Pekarek J et al "The clinical uses of specific transfer factors" in Recent Advances in Transfer factors and Dailyzable Leukocyte Extracts (1992) 256-63.
Pengelly A. "Medicinal fungi of the world" Modern Phytotherapist (1996)2:1,3–8.
Penn ND et al "The effect of dietary supplementation with vitamins A, C and E on cell-mediated immune function in elderly long-stay patients: a randomized controlled trial. Age Ageing (1991)20:169–74.

Pilotti V et al " Transfer factor as an adjuvant to non-small cell lung cancer" Biotherapy, (1996) 9(1-3): 117-121.

Pizza G et al "Effect of in vitro produced transfer factor on the immune response of cancer patients" European Journal of Cancer (1977) 13, 917-923.

Quinlan KP and Hayani KC "Vitamin A and respiratory syncytial virus infection" Serum levels and supplementation trial" Arch Pediatr Adolesc Med (1996)150:25–30.

Ringsdorf WM, et al "Sucrose, neutrophilic phagocytosis and resistance to disease" Dental Survey (1976)52(12):46.

Roda E et al "Transfer factor for the treatment of HbsAg-positive chronic active hepatitis. P. Soc. Exp. Med (1985) 178, 468-475.

Sacks N et al "The use of transfer factors in the treatment of multiple sclerosis: a case report" South Africa Medical Journal (1976 Sep 18) 50(40):1556-8.

Sanchez A et al "Role of sugars in human neutrophilic phagocytosis" American Journal of Clinical Nutrition (1973)26:1180.

Schulkind ML and Ayoub EM "Transfer factor and its clinical application" Advanced Pediatrics (1980) 27: 89-115.

Semba RD "Vitamin A and immunity to viral, bacterial and protozoan infections" Proc Nutr Soc (1999 Aug) 58(3):719-27.

Sibl O et al " The adjuvant therapy of nasopharyngeal tumor with transfer factor" in Research and Application of Transfer Factor and DLE (1989) 403-10.

Stallone DD "The influence of obesity and its treatment on the immune system" Nutrition Review (1994)52:37–50.

Steele RW et al "Transfer factor for the prevention of varicella-zoster infection in childhood leukemia" New.England Journal of Medicine (1980) 14; 303(7): 355-9.

Szabo G "Monocytes, alcohol use, and altered immunity" Alcohol Clin Exp Res (1998) 22:216–19S.

Tashiro T et al. "n-3 versus n-6 polyunsaturated fatty acids in critical illness" Nutrition (1998)14:551–3.

Valdimarsson H et al " Immune abnormalities associated with chronic mucocutaneous candidiasis" Cellular Immunology (1973) 6: 348.

Viza D et al "Orally administered specific transfer factor for the treatment of herpes infections" Lymphok Res (1985) 4, 27-30.

Viza D et al "Specific transfer factor protects mice against lethal challenge with herpes simplex virus" Cellular Immunity (1986) 100, 555-562.

Waddell C et al "Inhibition of lymphoproliferation by hyperlipoproteinemic plasma" Journal of Clinical Nutrition, (1976) 58: 950-54.

Watanabe H "Hepatitis C virus infection manifesting as tubulointerstitial nephritis, cardiomyopathy, and hepatitis" American Journal of Medicine (2000 Aug 1)109(2):176-7.

Whyte RI et al Adjuvant treatment using transfer factor for bronchogenic carcinoma: long-term follow-up" Annals of Thoracic Surgery (1992) 53(3): 391-6.

Wilson GB et al "Treatment of Mycobacterium-fortuitum pulmonary infection with Transfer Factor: New methodology for evaluating TF potency and predicting clincal response" Clinical Immunology and Immunopathology (1982) 23: 478.

Yaqoob P "Monounsaturated fats and immune function" Proc Nutr Soc (1998)57:511–20.

About the Author

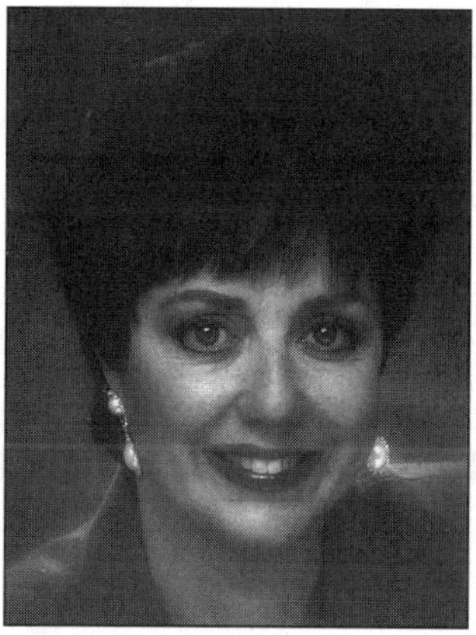

Rita Elkins, M.H., is the author of over 40 natural health titles, has written numerous magazine and other articles, and has been involved in the writing and production of various health reference materials. Her 15 years of investigating and covering natural health topics have made her a widely respected author in the health publishing world.

She is a regular contributor to *Let's Live* and *Great Life* magazines and has hosted radio talk shows on natural health topics. She lectures nationwide on the science behind natural compounds and collaborates with medical doctors on various projects. Her publications and lectures have been used by companies like Nature's Sunshine, 4-Life Research, Enrich, NuSkin, and Nutraceutical to support the credibility of natural supplementation. She has recently co-authored *Soy Smart Health* with the New York Times' Best Selling author Neil Solomon, MD.